MW01152934

The Mind Body Solution:

Train your Brain for Permanent Weight Loss

BY

AJ MIHRZAD M.S. CPT

DEDICATION

You know how it is. You pick up a book, flip to the dedication, and find that, once again, the author has dedicated a book to someone else and not to you.

Not this time...

This one's for you.

I'm proud of you for loving yourself and making your health a priority.

There's also a special place in my heart for caffeine which has been my companion through the long days of writing this book for you.

Let's get started, shall we?

TABLE OF CONTENTS

1/

NEAR DEATH: MY CRISIS

I was about to die. My heart felt like it was about to explode, and there was nothing that I could do about it. I froze at first, but then quickly knew that I had to fight for my life, or lose it *very* soon.

I had made a grave mistake: I had taken a huge drink of the wrong supplement, ingesting a toxic amount that was going right to my heart.

For many years, I had experimented with nutritional supplements in order to learn better and better ways to up my metabolism and burn more fat. Yes, I will admit it: this was motivated first by my own vanity. But I also truly wanted to help others to improve themselves. That was, before I realized that I was about to die. It was a gloomy, cloudy Saturday afternoon, and, in error I had inadvertently gulped down 3,000-times the recommended dose of Yohimbe HCl.

The moment that I swallowed the last bit of it, I suddenly realized what had happened. Frantic, I ran to the toilet and tried to vomit up what I had ingested by mistake. But nothing came out!!

At that point, I was already numb and certain that I was heading for death. Out of pure fear, I ran to my computer and Googled the "lethal dose" of this particular stimulant. Unfortunately, there were no ready answers as to how to reverse its effects.

I knew that I had only a few moments left to react and save my life, so I grabbed my little brother, and drove myself to the emergency room. As I staggered out of the car, I felt like my entire world was melting. Already racing, my heart beat furiously in my chest. I was sweating profusely and my eyeballs began to pop out of my skull.

I ran right straight into the ER, and forced my way up to the first doctor I saw. Grabbing his lab coat with all of the strength I had left, I blurted out that I was about to die.

I told him that I had taken an extreme amount of fat burner by accident, and that I only had minutes to live before my heart would explode.

He reacted in a very logical way. First, he told me to calm down. I'm sure he thought that I was just high on some drug, and surely overreacting.

Then, he handed me a clipboard with some forms, and asked me to follow the hospital's procedures and fill them out.

I tried … but I quickly started to fade in and out of consciousness.

I had barely written anything on the form when I felt the pen drop from my hand. Then, I blacked out.

When I regained consciousness, I was surrounded by doctors and nurses. In that moment, my life literally flashed before my eyes.

I remembered everything that had happened in my entire life: my birthdays, graduating from high school, my first car, and even the first time I kissed a girl. I remembered the many times that I had looked at myself in the mirror, overweight and depressed, and felt disgusted about my appearance.

That seemed to be the reason why I was dying. Then, I passed out again.

I had another flash where I saw my family crying: my parents and brothers sobbing. I heard the doctor say to them that I wasn't going to make it, that my heart rate had been over 180 beats per minute for the past three days.

"He's not going to live." I heard it plainly.

All that time, I had been in a coma and heavily sedated. My body fought against my overdose for dear life, trying to clear out of my system enough stimulant to kill a horse.

Finally, on the fourth day, I woke up with tubes coming out of all different parts of my body. I had a breathing device and a catheter inside (I shudder to think about how they inserted *those* in my body). When I could speak, I asked my mom what had happened.

It turns out that I had spent five days in a coma. Just as I had thought, I had nearly died. In fact, I **did** die, but then, I came back to life.

My heart rate, which had spiked to 180 beats per minute in response to my ingesting so much stimulant/fat-burner, miraculously dropped back down to normal after about four days. By Thursday, it felt like just yesterday that I drank the wrong bottle of supplement mix. All of a sudden, everything started to make sense.

After surviving that incident, I began to question a lot of things about my life and where it was going. One week after returning home from the hospital, I went into a deep depression, full of self-loathing. I really got down on myself for almost dying just because I was so desperate to be thin. Not only was that the lowest point of my life, it was also a major turning point for me.

That near-death experience made me realize how short my life could have been. Imagine:

AJ Mihrzad: Died in 2006 trying to lose weight.

I've suffered from being overweight most of my life, and now I had almost killed myself trying to be thin. That was when I realized that I had to do something, not just for myself, but to help others as well. This is what you're going to learn in this book. It's what led me to leave my legacy.

2/

MY AMAZING FITNESS SUCCESS

Having been overweight for most of my life, I know personally what it's like to be out of shape. It wasn't until I hit rock bottom, however, that I actually did something about it.

On the day that I turned my life around, I walked out of a McDonald's, looked over, and saw my chubby profile reflected back at me in the front window. I stopped in my tracks because I couldn't believe what I saw. I had totally let myself go. I was shocked and disgusted. No matter how hard I tried, I couldn't hide the layers of fat that covered my body.

My clothes didn't even fit me right; they looked silly on me. In fact, I had a whole closet that was full of clothes no longer my size.

I felt the burden of all that extra weight like iron chains of fat that were limiting me from living my true life. I looked like I didn't care about either myself or my health. It appeared that I sat around all day, eating junk and processed foods, not caring one damn bit about the way I looked.

But seriously, *I DID care*.

On that one particular late-summer evening, I became really distraught and disappointed with myself. I went home, climbed upstairs to my dark room, and fell into bed. Then, as I lay there in deep depression and sadness, I had this newfound **Revelation.** At that very moment I felt an immense rush of emotional pain. I decided that I'd finally had enough.

Right at that moment, I swore this to myself: "I am going to get into the best SHAPE of my LIFE!!"

The feeling was so intense and my mind was so clear that I knew I had to give myself that chance to get my life back.

At first, though, I didn't even know how to go about getting into shape. I was undecided about joining a gym. I told some of my friends at work about my mission, and they all actually laughed at me.

"You? Be healthy and get in shape?? *In Your Dreams*!! Ha Ha Ha!"

Their comments upset me deep to my core, and reconfirmed my feelings of hopelessness.

Having my own friends say such things also made me angry. So I used that anger to bring me back to that day of my revelation. I **_had_** to stop dead in my tracks, and **_cease_** such negative and irrational thoughts about myself in order to take even the very first steps.

So, instead, I began to tell myself this: "I am not hopeless. I matter!!"

And with that, I dragged myself down to the gym and worked out for hours on end. I didn't even know what I was doing, at first! I pushed, I pulled, and I even grunted a few times. But after all that work, I achieved only minimal results.

Along with the initial exercise, I also tried all kinds of expensive fat-burning pills that were supposed to increase my metabolic rate and kill my cravings. In fact, they did nothing but make me feel panicky and jittery.

I went on zero-carb diets as well, but they made me crave sugar so much that I pigged out on high carbs and sweet binges. Afterwards, the guilt destroyed my motivation.

I tried another fad diet that involved eating and drinking only protein shakes and protein bars. Unfortunately, they made me so hungry; I became as ravenous as an emaciated lion in the desert.

I ordered workout DVD's and video tapes. You should have seen me try to follow along with them in my living room. It was a joke! And soon, the boredom and lack of motivation made the whole attempt unbearable. No wonder NOBODY gets results with those things.

I then invested in a home gym. I bought gym equipment, machines, free weights, push-up bars and cardio equipment. But they were soon collecting cobwebs and taking up all of my free space, becoming expensive hangers for my clothes.

Believe me, I tried everything imaginable. Nothing worked for me.

Deep in my gut, though, I knew that there had to be something more to it. Something that I was missing. Something that I was doing wrong.

I became determined to find out what that was.

I even took drastic measures. First, I enrolled in college, and majored in Exercise Science and Nutrition. I purchased every text book, magazine, and product available that involved fitness and nutrition. I was determined to find the cure for my problem.

I literally spent hundreds of hours studying on the internet, along with taking college courses and text book reading. Instead of consuming food, I consumed every functional piece of information that I could get my hands on. I studied, I applied the things that worked for me, and I dismissed those that didn't. Night after night I stayed up until sunrise, trying to figure out the perfect, quickest fat-loss program. I discovered that there was a lot of propaganda out there, and that finding the truth was like searching for the Holy Grail.

What I discovered surprised me...

As I spent so much time researching and studying everything related to exercise and nutrition, I realized that there was one component that had to be mastered, as well.

That missing link was the **mind**. I was compelled next to learn about the inner workings of the human mind, so I went back to graduate school and got my Master's degree in psychology.

As I completed my Master's, I also read every book and article that I could get my hands on about mental training. I was reading 2-3 books a week on the subjects of exercise, nutrition, and psychology, easily.

As I delved deeper into this learning process, I discovered that there are **Three Pillars to Fitness**. I set out to create the perfect weight-loss program that encompasses all three.

I basically stumbled onto the secrets and lies that the so-called "experts" in the fat-loss industry *don't want you to know .*

When most people try to get into shape, they rely on advice that is given in popular books, magazines and fitness websites ... This is a HUGE problem.

Let me explain.

The Fat-Loss Industry is a Big, Big Business, and the competition within it is vicious. This year alone, Americans spent over $60 billion on fad diets, shakes, dietary supplements, and fat-loss programs. Everyone wants a piece of that, and will fight for it in the most devious ways.

Fact 1: The diet and weight-loss industry is so loosely regulated that huge corporations that dominate it get away with highway robbery.

Fact 2: Many of the popular fitness magazines and websites are owned by major nutrition and dietary supplement companies. So a lot of the information published in these periodicals is nothing but sneaky ads for their products.

Fact 3: The same companies allocate tons of funds towards marketing, including the purchase of expensive television and newspaper ads, in order to spin the "news" any which way they want to present it.

So, what you're reading and watching about weight loss on the news is usually NOTHING more than what these large corporations want you to believe.

I'm sorry to be the one to bring you the Truth ... But!

You have been lied to by these Greedy Weight Loss corporations Over and Over again. Because of all this dishonesty, most people who try to lose fat are doing it incorrectly.

People rely on bland foods, powders, and "magical drinks." They use the wrong exercises, follow ineffective workouts, and do even worse in their attempts to lose weight ...

In fact, when most people exercise, their form is actually *hazardous* to their health!

Not only are these mistakes highly unproductive; they can also cause permanent injures to your body. You may damage or destroy your joints and ligaments, plus end up with crooked posture. (Observe the population at any gym, and you'll see what I mean.)

So, what did I do once I had uncovered all of these deceptions and ruthless strategies?

I Got Revenge. The *best* kind possible, in fact: I got into mind-blowing shape without relying on their <u>lies</u> and - <u>inferior products</u>!

So what was my **Game plan**?

I created the **most effective and fastest muscle-toning and fat-burning strategy possible,** based on all of my collective knowledge and experience.

What do you think happened???

The ugly fat literally **melted off** my body. Muscles that I never knew I had become hard and defined.

In total, I lost 53 pounds, and got into the BEST SHAPE OF MY LIFE...

Barely **anyone** *believed that I could transform myself, but I truly DID!*

And that's just the start. I now feel like I'm 10 years younger than my actual age, and I have incredible energy. I even stand prouder and taller.

Also, my immune system became very strong; I haven't gotten sick in years, and feel terrific all day long!

But the most exciting aspect of my transformation was what happened to my self-image. Now, when I look in the mirror, I'm pretty damn grateful for what I see. My social life is better. My relationships are better. My well-being is better. In fact, EVERYTHING has improved.

Now, my story could've ended there, but for me, it was only the beginning. In fact, it became even more exciting: *I became the most wanted Fitness Guru on Long Island!*

As I continued to look better and better, something really <u>strange</u> began to happen. People constantly asked me questions, like:

"How did you lose ALL that fat so fast?" and

"What do you do to look SO good?" and

"Can you help ME look better too?"

People practically BEGGED me to help them get in amazing shape. I did give them a few pointers here and there, but without putting much thought into it.

Still … guess what happened?!?

The very first person whom I helped, he lost 27 pounds in less than 8 weeks. The next person lost 49 pounds in just 4 months!!

And these were just the *first two people* that I had EVER helped.

I was brand new to this whole fitness/nutrition/mind thing; I just did it for FUN. I had certainly never before had people beg me for information about how to change *their* habits, or *how to live better.* Those initial successes made me realize, though, just how much I enjoyed changing people's lives!

Soon thereafter, I <u>knew</u> what my passion was. I discovered what it was that I wanted to do with my life.

I wanted to help other people <u>look good</u> and <u>feel</u> <u>great!</u>

At the time, I still had some reservations, however, about going into the personal training and weight loss business, because I had friends who'd had horrible experiences with personal trainers when they'd tried to get in shape. They described to me their many bad experiences with personal trainers, paying their hard-earned money but not seeing any results.

My friends described typical work-out sessions where their trainer would just hold a clipboard as they yapped away about their own personal lives. These personal trainers also rarely seemed to understand human physiology or basic nutrition concepts.

I discovered that, when people hired a personal trainer, their major issue was being coached to do the same tedious workout routine over and over again. (Your body adapts rapidly to the same movements; you need a variety of exercises in order to make improvements.)

I was disgusted to learn the many negative experiences connected with traditional personal trainers. But I decided that, just because there were some spoiled eggs in the industry, that wouldn't stop me. In fact, it fired me up. I decided to use those complaints to my benefit, and set a positive example for other trainers to follow.

When I was in college studying Exercise Science and Nutrition, my first job was at a local corporate gym training members. You know these types of places: they are advertised on national television. After a short time I found myself so aggravated that the gym management was more focused on sales rather than on their clients' fitness results. All of us trainers were told to focus on selling packages, as opposed to getting people in optimal shape. Our managers had us hard-sell memberships, along with useless dietary pills and shakes. I was soon beside myself with aggravation, and got into several altercations with my supervisors around these issues. This was *not* what I had set out to do.

I quickly figured out that, if I wanted to live my passion and help people get into mind-blowing shape, I needed to use my own unique knowledge and abilities to stop a speeding freight train dead in its tracks. I had to break away from the prevailing fitness-industry standards. So I put all of my education, knowledge, and experience together, and created the "LifeFuelFit Program," my very own fitness program.

The "LifeFuelFit Program" is the fastest and most effective method for transforming the human body. It is not just a cutting-edge routine that improves the physical body; it also enhances the way the mind works to support health and fitness.

I was able to help countless people get the bodies they yearned for rapidly. I helped every person who crossed my path. Shortly after founding my unique program, the demand for my services literally shot through the roof!

What really amazed me was that most of the people I trained **never** thought that they could have a great body or feel so awesome. In a blink of an eye, though, I was able to get them into a leaner, more toned shape. Even their own family members didn't recognize them without doing a double take.

As a result of so many night-and-day transformations, it wasn't long before the waiting list for my services grew **far** beyond what I was able to handle, myself.

So here's what I did. I systematized the "LifeFuelFit Program," and hired a team of highly qualified and top results-producing trainers and nutritionists in my local area. These are TRULY the cream of the crop, and they use the exact same training systems that have been proven to work for my clients time and again.

Here's why this program works so well:

As I mentioned, I've personally been overweight and out of shape, and have less than average genetics. My program takes an approach that diverges radically from that of genetically-blessed trainers who've been in good shape all of their lives, those who believe that what works for them definitely works for everyone.

My program is for people with "less than average" genetics.

What we do is to **blend cutting-edge, proven scientific strategies with fun and innovative state-of-the-art exercise techniques** that transform your body literally overnight.

We also apply the right state of mind: high-energy, top-notch motivation partnered with world-class guidance, experienced instruction, and total support. This workout experience delivers exceptional results. The bottom line is that you're going to **look amazing**, no matter what kind of genes you were born with.

We frequently change-up your program so that you never get bored to death with the same routine. You will make non-stop progress because you won't be able to adapt to the various methods. My system literally "tricks" your body into peak shape.

To find out more about my transformation program, you can go to my website www.LifeFuelFit.com.

3/

MY METHOD

I'm going to share methods that others may charge thousands of dollars for. I am going to give you **the exact strategy** for how I helped hundreds of people get into the best shape of their lives! Rather than go into every intricate aspect of the programs, however, I will cover how much your **mind affects your fitness goals**.

"Unconscious eating" is the number one cause of obesity today. The one fact—and the biggest lesson—that I've learned as a fitness professional is this: if we eat without thinking about it, we are going to

- ➢ eat the wrong foods,
- ➢ eat too much food, and
- ➢ become overweight as a result of it.

This is called "mindless eating." I found that the clearer your mind, the more conscious you are. The more conscious, the better you are going to follow any solid fitness program.

As you know by now, I struggled with being overweight for many years; I tried numerous diets and workout plans to no avail. Nothing ever helped me as much as what I'm going to share with you.

One of the major insights that I came across was the fact that all of us are constantly **thinking erratically**. Our minds are all over the place. We think about the past, or we worry about the future constantly. We have approximately 60,000 thoughts per day, and the majority of them are useless and repetitive. In fact, many of them are negative.

The scary thing is that <u>**our thoughts are making us fat!**</u> In his *New York* Times best-selling diet book, "Why We Get Fat," acclaimed science writer Gary Taubes discusses how just the fact of our **thinking about carbohydrates** raises our insulin levels and causes fat gain. We are getting more obese not by eating ... Just By THINKING!

These thoughts also cloud our true selves because, in reality, all we have is <u>this moment</u>. Right now, as you're reading the words on this page, <u>that</u> is all we have. **This moment!**

Billions of bits of information compete against or for our attention. So, many times, we aren't focusing on the right things. But these thoughts, feelings, and emotions do cause us to overeat.

In addition, we also rationalize about why we're not exercising. We're in a state of "busy." *Everybody* is busy.

When I ask my clients, "Why aren't you working out as often?" their answer is, "because I'm too busy."

I ask, "Why aren't you eating healthy foods?"

Their answer is, "because they take too long to prepare and I don't have the time."

These are merely limiting beliefs. As we proceed together, I will <u>shatter</u> all of these limiting beliefs that hold you back from health and fitness.

"A person can live 40 days without food, 4 days without water, 4 minutes without air, but only 4 seconds without Hope."—John Maxwell

Nick Sisman worked on a train crew. It seemed like Nick had everything that a man could want: a wife, two healthy children, a decent job, and many friends.

However, Nick had one fault. He was a notorious worrier. He worried about everything, and usually feared the worst.

One midsummer day, the train crew was informed that they could quit an hour early in honor of the foreman's birthday. Accidentally, when the rest of the workmen left the site, Nick was locked in a refrigerator boxcar.

Nick panicked! He banged and shouted until his fists were bloody and his voice was hoarse. No one heard him.

"If I can't get out, I'll freeze to death in here," he thought. Wanting to let his wife and family know exactly what had happened to him, Nick found a knife and began to etch words on the wooden floor.

He wrote:

"It's so cold, my body is getting numb. If I could just go to sleep, these may be my last words..."

The next morning, when the crew slid open the heavy doors of the boxcar, they found Nick dead. An autopsy revealed that every physical sign in his body indicated that he had frozen to death, yet the refrigeration unit of the car was inoperative, and the temperature inside never fell below a mild fifty-five degrees!

Crazy, right?

This story teaches me that "The Mind is Powerful."

The mind is so powerful that it can convince you of things that are just not true.

I found a scientific study that explains how the mind affects the ways that our body gains and loses weight. The study discusses how a specific thinking pattern can actually make you leaner. What this means is that **you may currently be thinking thoughts that make you FAT!!**

Alternately, just being <u>conscious</u> of the fact that you are exercising *can* lead to better fitness!

In February 2007, a study published by Harvard University in *Psychological Science* tracked the health of 84 female room attendants who worked in several different hotels. The researchers found that women who recognized their work as "exercise" experienced significant health benefits.

The women were separated into two groups.

One group was told that their daily work actually fulfilled all of their recommended daily requirements healthy activity levels. The other women, the "control group," went about their work as usual without the benefit of that information.

Although neither group changed their behavior, in just four weeks the women who were conscious of their activity level experienced a significant drop in weight, blood pressure, body fat, waist-to-hip ratio, and body mass index.

The "control group" experienced no health improvements, despite their engaging in the same physical activities.

This study illustrates the profound ways in which a person's attitude can affect their physical well-being.

It's amazing that just being conscious of the fact that you are involved in a transformation program—only a slight shift in your thinking—can yield profound results!

World-renowned psychologist Abraham Maslow created his own "hierarchy of needs." Within this framework, he identified the core needs of all human beings. Unless a specific primary need is fulfilled, a person can never get to their next need. The theory is very simple, and clearly defined in Maslow's profound study, where he delves into these needs individually:

► Food

► Shelter

► Love

► Family, and the last one,

► Self-Actualization

In a similar way, you are not going to reach your health and fitness goals unless you have taken care of these basic needs.

This is where the mental aspects of weight loss and fitness come into play. Unless you are mentally sound and everything is aligned, you will not be able to focus on your fitness and health with the same sense of insight that you can, once those needs are fully met.

So, make sure to keep that in mind. **First, you must take care of the inner game and be fully focused, in tune with yourself. Then—and only once you are at one and at peace with yourself—you can utilize the powerful principals of mindful eating.**

That statement is very profound.

I'm going to detail many powerful tactical insights that will help you to accomplish ideal health. I will teach you many of the same type of insights, and show you, first hand, how to apply them to your fitness goals.

Our bodies consist of three things:

- ▶ what we eat,
- ▶ what we drink, and
- ▶ what we think.

Thinking, or our psychology, is a very important part of our fitness.

Ask yourself this question: why are there no obese wild animals? The only animals that are obese are either domesticated or captive in a zoo. In other words, the fat animals are those that are mainly around humans.

The reasons for their obesity are:

1. **Wild animals have a natural mechanism to stop eating** when full. When a domesticated animal like a dog

lives in close proximity to humans, it will eat even though it's full. It will continue to eat, vomit, and then eat some more.

2. **Wild animals are always in the present moment**. They lack a frontal lobe, so they do not live in their thoughts. They do not think of the past or the future. They are always present, clear-minded, and attuned to their intuition about their natural satiety. Only domesticated animals become overweight. Dogs and cats take on the unconscious eating habits of their owners. A cluttered mind equals emotional eating. People who have cluttered minds tend to be more impulsive in their eating habits.

3. **Animals are in the wild**. Our ancestors used to be outdoors, as well, and moved around constantly. Now, we are imprisoned by our own technology. We stay indoors and burn much fewer calories. This trend is only getting worse.

I want to talk about our **true essence:** happiness, and how it relates to weight loss.

Happiness is the elusive feeling that everybody seeks. I used to focus only on being happy, and tried to chase after it. My being depressed and overweight for so long exacerbated a sense that something was missing from my life. I had deep feelings that something was wrong with me because I was so depressed and down on myself. I was overweight at the time, too, and believed that my many negative thoughts were limiting factors that had really slowed down my life.

Here is the story of an embarrassing example, but one where I began to realize that I had **self-limiting beliefs**. It is about my first kiss.

It came totally out of the blue. I was, in fact, kissed by one of my friends. It all happened one day in high school when I was alone with her in a classroom, working on a project. I was minding my own business when, all of a sudden, she put her face in front of mine. I paused, a bit shocked.

Then, out of nowhere, she started to kiss me. I did <u>not</u> know what to do! As I tried to coordinate my tongue with hers, I ended up licking her nose and chin! It was a funny moment; I woke up and said, "Wow: somebody finds me attractive." (That was back when I thought that I was the ugliest person on the face of the earth.)

Growing up, in fact, I had *always* thought that I was ugly. I was sure that my face was really unattractive, and that lowered my confidence and made me very shy. Once, in seventh grade, a girl pointed to me and said, in front of all her friends, "Oh my God, that's the ugliest person in the world." And they all laughed.

Sadly, I believed her. It bothered me for many years.

My being overweight for so much of my life led me to have a great deal of insecurity about my body, too. Even though I lost close to 50 pounds and put myself into fantastic physical shape, I continued to deal with many of the same psychological issues that I had when I was overweight. That goes to show how little I valued myself, and how little others valued me. I still see that ugly, chubby boy sometimes, even though many people have told me to become a paid model.

Insecurities never fully go away. When I was overweight, I dealt with three main things. They still haunt me until this day. One was my big chipmunk cheeks, because being overweight led me to have a moon face. Second was my man boobs, which always poked out of my shirt and were super embarrassing, even with my clothes on. Third, of course, was my big old fat gut.

It's funny because, right now as I walk around, I'm sporting a six-pack. My body fat is at 8%. But still, the moment I slip on my diet or I feel like I'm retaining some water, I always notice the fat gain in my trouble areas. My face gets bloated, my nipples get puffy, and I feel like I have chest fat, plus my stomach feels like it is protruding.

I guess that will never go away. In life, we just have to deal with our insecurities, and live in spite of them.

Logically, I know that I'm a decent-looking guy, and that I have a fit body. However, I still have a hard time looking in the mirror and seeing the fitness model that others see when they look at me. And I'm ok with that, it keeps me humble.

Even thinking a crazy, irrational thought like being the ugliest person was just a figment of my imagination. It was an *irrational thought* that I came to believe, but when my high school friend reached over and kissed me, all of a sudden, it washed away. I find times like that really interesting, when something happens that shatters your limitations.

As I grew older and continued to live those negative patterns, my depression became worse. I ran them over and over in my mind, and became more and more angry. These thoughts even led me to do things that were very irrational, because I developed access to more ways to injure or destroy myself.

In my early twenties, for example, I started to experiment with drugs and alcohol. I literally tried to find happiness through substances. For many years, I experimented with just about every drug known to mankind, trying to feel some level of happiness. When I reached it, I'd feel great, and then, suddenly, come crashing down and become depressed for days afterwards.

I lived on this emotional roller coaster for many years. It led me to gain even more weight, and be even more self-destructive. Clearly, I was trying to find something that didn't exist. But I kept looking for some sort of happiness, traveling along the pathways of drugs and alcohol that were slowly killing me. It wasn't until I had some really dark moments that I opened my eyes. It was experiences with extreme drugs that nearly led to my demise. Trying to find happiness through food and toxic substances caused my obesity. Self-destructive behaviors almost killed me.

I am very thankful that I'm alive today, and that I don't do that crap anymore. In reality, it taught me a lot, so I don't regret anything that I went through; it became part of my motivation to write this book, and relive those dark, terrible, sad moments of my life. The self-destructive behaviors did make me realize that, if I continued to seek happiness through external sources—whether through relationships, drugs or food—then I was headed down a horrible path in life.

I've never believed in reincarnation. I can't see myself coming back as a slug. That doesn't vibe too well with me. I believe that reincarnation symbolizes being born again in the moment. Simply changing your thoughts allows you to reincarnate into a new person. I'm completely different than I was 10 years ago. In fact, a decade ago, I was one big mess. I used to be overweight, pessimistic, and insecure; I had really low expectations.

Now, I'm a completely different person, and I've worked hard to improve myself in every aspect. I also know that, 10 years from now, I'll change even more!

The atoms that make up everything on earth are the same atoms that have been used over and over again to make everything for the last 4.6 billion years. We lose and regenerate many cells on a daily basis: every 7 days, a new version of us is formed.

We evolve thought by thought. Our mind is constantly creating stories that make us hate, suffer, and hurt ourselves. By the same token, our mind can be used to love, give, and inspire.

In a split second, you could devolve into a lower version of yourself, or evolve to a higher version. It's all about the thoughts that YOU choose: they lead you towards your destined path.

"The mind can make a heaven out of hell or a hell out of heaven"

—John Milton

I truly believe that, at this very moment, we can reincarnate into the *greatest* version of ourselves and create the life of our dreams…

Then again, I may be wrong, and come back as a slug. Giving up salt would really suck. I'd much rather be a monkey. Not the ones with the red butt-cheeks, though.

4/

MAXIMIZING THIS MOMENT

As you subtract all of the negative and toxic things in your life, you will allow the truly vital things to flourish. Then, you can focus your time, energy, and willpower on the most important goal: living healthier. Without your health, nothing else matters. When a person is sick, how can they care about how much money they have, or how many other material items? If their life is in danger and fading by the moment, they can't. It is sad to say but, when a person is near death, sometimes only then do they really embrace every moment and cherish each breath. All of a sudden, they're put up against a deadline.

When people are near death and they know that their time on earth is limited, they come to realize what is truly important. On the other hand, when we are healthy, we often believe that we have an abundance of time.

The pressing concept of time can also be a burden; we may feel that we aren't where we "need" to be in life. These expectations can cause us to think that bad things are going to happen, and lead us to invent worrying mental stories. This pattern of negative thinking creates unnecessary stress that is toxic to our livelihood.

I want to take you back to the point of **simply focusing in on the moment**. This is all that you have, after all. I have found that the more you live in the moment, the better your choices are going to be, and the less you're going to allow your erratic thinking to control the path of your life. You're going to make better choices, and have a sense of clarity and happiness.

I can sum up my philosophy simply: "**Maximize This Moment.**" That is at the core of my Mind-Body Solution. If you keep that as a mantra and live by it, then all is well. Of course, it's not so easy as to just adopt a mantra and repeat it; actually living it is a different matter. In reality, it takes time and effort, just like anything in life.

You may ask, what does "maximizing the moment" have to do with losing weight and achieving optimal health?

I've found that a lot of people who have exercised and tried every diet plan around *still* have trouble losing weight. I taught them to maximize the moment, and implement my Mind-Body Solution. It has helped them, and that's why I can help you.

I believe that, once you are able to abide by this principle, and apply it to your life along with the other ideas that I share in this book, not only are you going to lose weight, feel healthier, and be more vibrant with energy, but you're also going to achieve a level of happiness and peace of mind that you've never felt before.

When I was younger, I used to chase happiness as if I were missing out on something. As though, if I weren't happy, something was wrong with me. Boy, was that a mistake!

Once you've discovered being in the present moment, and then focus on taking a lot of things *out* of your life—literally subtracting them—you will feel more at peace. From a larger point of view, you're going to have an abundance of time, and also decrease the feeling of "need" in your life.

With peace of mind, you're going to become more disciplined and in control because, if you look at the deeper level of why a person is overweight, it connects to their lack of self-control. They lack control over their eating. They don't know when to stop. They allow their emotions to, in a sense, guide them to what they should eat and to what makes them feel good. They *don't* have the control within themselves to go to the gym, or to perform cardio.

Lack of control is what is sabotaging their life. I'm sure that this lack of control is also present in other areas, as well. One of the main focuses of this book is to show you how to gain control. It all starts with controlling this moment, controlling your life right NOW, and controlling that which you have power over. The more you control this moment, the more you will control your life as a whole.

With the decisions you make, you become connected to this moment, and no longer controlled by the random currents of life. I'm going to go deeply into some strategies to make you realize this. It's not about teaching theories, though: I believe in actually giving you action steps that you can use to make dramatic changes in your life.

One of the biggest things that I've realized is that we're always trying to add "things" into our life. We have this belief that, if we add certain things, we'll get happier as a result. I've come to find the opposite! *You will become happier when you subtract certain things out of your life*, because then, you can focus on the important key factors in your life that will help you to improve it.

Think of it like this: you must simplify in order to multiply.

It starts with your thinking. As I mentioned, we have 60,000 thoughts per day. If you subtract 10% of them, you will have 10% fewer unnecessary thoughts to cause you emotional turmoil, or make you do things mindlessly. All of a sudden, you're going to see a dramatic improvement in your life. When you separate from current negative habits or toxic relationships, you free yourself from the time and energy that you used to devote to disempowering factors that hold you back. You lose what I think of as energy-suckers and time-vampires, in the greatest sense.

You also subtract things that you've been doing, whether they are activities or certain obligations, which you don't need to do anymore. All of a sudden you will create more time for yourself, because you won't be doing useless activities that used to take up time.

A great example of this is how you treat your finances. The reason why America is in a debt crisis is because people have the tendency to buy certain things in order to add more than they need. Americans spend more money than they have in order to achieve joy. I believe that if, instead, they did the opposite, and got rid of things, they'd have more money and more happiness.

"The smaller the area of focus, the greater the mind's clarity'"

—Anonymous

Time is the enemy of the mind. What I mean by that is this: we get stressed because we have certain goals or want certain things to happen, and they don't, within the timeframe that we imagine.

When we look at time, we're thinking about our own life and comparing it to others'. We're saying to ourselves: "in this time I should be married," "I should have kids," "I should be a millionaire," and so on. It's not until we take the time to look at it that we realize, this is a figment of our imagination.

The present moment is all there is. When you take away time, all of a sudden you will have an abundance of it to do with as you please. The reality is this: we are all unique in our own way, and we're going to reach our specific milestones when the right time comes. There is no specific deadline for things to happen and, whether they happen or not, we are still going to be fine.

That is basically the premise of being in the moment, and enjoying the moment because you're enjoying the ride. You're not looking towards the end-point or the destination, and thinking, "once I'm at the destination, that's when I'll be happy."

Why not enjoy every moment that leads you to the destination? That is one of the biggest things that has helped me because I try to stay as present as I possibly can. There are a lot of things that I employ to stay present and focused. I'm going to share these things throughout the course of this book. But first, I want to emphasize the simple premise of living in the moment, enjoying it, and thinking about how you can "maximize" it.

What are the things around you or opportunities that you feel, deep down in your gut, that you should be doing?

Keeping this in mind, most of our thoughts are unnecessary and incessant. They do more harm than good. In order to reach a higher level of happiness and gain more clarity in your life, simply reduce the amount of thinking throughout your day. This can be done in many ways.

You should focus on reducing your thoughts, being in the present moment, and giving your attention to what's important and towards thoughts that empower you. Whatever the present moment presents to you, you should make the best out of it—capitalize on it in order to fit it into your bigger picture.

All you have in life is a series of moments. Life is not the past nor is it the future. It is happening as you read these words in front of you. As you read this, your life is unfolding. So, why should you allow your thoughts and anxieties to ruin this amazing aspect of your life, which is unfolding as we speak?

I lost my phone one morning. I searched for an hour and ransacked my entire house. I still couldn't find it.

I panicked. Not so much for the phone itself; more so for the incriminating pictures and the volumes of personal notes that I had saved on it. They are irreplaceable and embarrassing, if ever shown in the light of day. God forbid they end up in the wrong hands.

After I made my house look like a burglar had fumbled through it, I went to my neighbor's house and asked her to call my phone. My urgent knock abruptly woke her up. She greeted me wearing a tie-died Mumu, and a look on her face that would make a baby cry in terror.

She proceeded to dial my number. A few seconds later, I felt my right butt cheek vibrating. Sheepishly, I pulled out my phone from my back pocket, and gave ole meanie an awkward smile.

As I walked back home, something occurred to me…

I've been feeling really good as of late, and was trying to figure out, why this was so?

That little tremble on my ass muscle gave me a major insight!

I stopped looking for happiness.

Instead, I focused on peace of mind, and happiness came in through the back door.

You see, I used to search for happiness through external sources, whether it was illegal substances, alcohol, toxic relationships, or materialistic things.

Sure, those things made me happy, but it was short-lived and it fleeted fast. Soon after, I would feel empty and alone, oftentimes even worse than I had felt before the temporary moment of joy.

Every time that I looked outward for my high, shortly after, I felt the low.

It wasn't until I stopped chasing the highs that, instead, they started to look for me. I've come to discover that everything in life comes to you when you don't look for it.

Stop searching for money, love, and happiness. Allow it to find you.

The key is not to look outward, but rather to look inward. Inner peace is within your grasp at all times. All you need to do is look inside your heart to find it.

No matter what the outside circumstances are--whether you are angry, anxious, sad or scared--look inside to find your place of peace, and surrender to whatever is going on.

Wishing it were better only makes it worse. Be at peace with where you are. Even if you're feeling shitty, feel the emotion and embrace it.

SCREAM! CRY! RUN around the block a few times!

Let it out.

Let it pass.

To not feel your emotions is to be void of life.

As soon as you experience it, return back to your place of peace: your home, the place where happiness exists and emanates from.

It's your true essence. Everything else is secondary. If you're able to breath, then you can tap into that bliss.

Yes you're going to pass through storms, that's a given. But remember: no matter how volatile the sky is, when your rise above the dark clouds, there's a place of peace and serenity.

A place called space. Space exists above the clouds and inside you.

Tap into your inner space, and get High off your own Supply...

The next time you search for something, make sure that you don't already have it within you.

5/

INHALE/EXHALE

One thing that I do every day, in order to get focused in the present moment, is a simple breathing exercise. I do this each morning plus again at night, sometimes, when my thoughts are running out of control. If I'm having a stressful day, I'll do it a few times throughout the day as well, just to bring myself back and help me to stay grounded. This simple exercise involves counting from one to a hundred, while focusing on every breath.

You just inhale through the nose, and then exhale through the mouth, inhale on one, exhale on two, inhale counting three, exhale counting four, and so on and so forth, until you reach 100. When I first started to do this, it was very challenging. By the time I had counted to 20, my thoughts were all over the place, so it was very difficult to reach 100 for some time. But the more that I practiced it, the easier it got. Now, I do it every morning, first thing. Some may call it meditation; others look at it as a simple counting exercise. For me, it gives immense benefit.

Why? Because I'm in the present moment. Counting to 100 gives the exercise a logical start and ending. It's kind of like running. Some people can just put on their jogging shoes and run for hours on end. Me, I hate running—I prefer to use a treadmill with a timer, so I know when to stop.

Do what suits you best. If you want to focus on your breathing and meditate, then go for that. If you want to count only as high as 20 that's fine too. Do whatever you can every morning to calm your mind before beginning the day.

To practice deep breathing, inhale through your nose and exhale through your mouth. Remember to:

- Breathe more slowly
- Breathe more deeply, from the belly
- Exhale longer than you inhale.

Keep in mind that there is no "right way" to do this. I like to call my breathing exercise "taking ME time." Whatever we call it—mediation, prayer, or even solitude—it all serves the same purpose. It allows us to take some time during each day to observe our thoughts and clear our mind. When we spend a tiny amount of time being more aware and less distracted, our lives improve exponentially.

Deep breathing is not only relaxing: it's been scientifically proven to affect the heart, the brain, digestion, the immune system—and maybe even the expression of genes.

The relaxation response is controlled by another set of nerves, the main one being the **Vagus nerve**. Think of a car throttling down the highway at 120 miles an hour. That's the stress response. The Vagus nerve is the brake. When you are stressed, you have your foot on the gas, pedal to the floor. When you take slow, deep breaths, that is like engaging the brake.

Most important, this breathing exercise reduces your cortisol levels. **Cortisol** is the stress hormone, and it's just as nasty as it sounds. As if you didn't have enough problems already, it will make you store fat around your middle like a spare tire.

Cortisol is a hormone that is secreted by the adrenal glands. It regulates blood pressure, along with the body's use of macronutrients. Cortisol also affects the release of insulin, and your body's ability to convert sugars into energy.

Typically, cortisol levels peak in the morning, and are at their lowest levels in the middle of the night. At natural healthy levels, cortisol provides your body with sustained energy, and even improves memory. In stressful situations, however, extra cortisol is released in order to give the body an immediate, easy-to-use energy supply. While this reaction is helpful in life-or-death situations, it actually becomes harmful when it occurs in response to minor everyday stresses like traffic and bills. Chronic stress, over-working, and insufficient sleep cause a chronic excess of cortisol, which is harmful in the short-term, and life-threatening in the long-term.

Most modern-day stresses are mental or emotional—not truly life-threatening. The result of a week's worth of minor conflicts is a body under constant stress. This results in a few immediate complications:

▶ Suppressed thyroid function
▶ Lowered immune response
▶ Imbalanced blood sugar

Over the course of a lifetime, excess cortisol is associated with far more damaging effects:

▶ Loss of muscle mass, which also slows your metabolism.
▶ Chronically elevated blood sugar levels, which increase appetite and cravings for harmful sweets, and can lead to insulin resistance (a precursor of type 2 diabetes).

▶ Accumulation of body fat from "stress eating" due to an over stimulated appetite. "Stress eating" tends to add fat around the abdomen. Belly fat is linked to metabolic syndrome: a group of risk factors correlated with increased incidence of type-2 diabetes, heart disease, obesity, high cholesterol, and high blood pressure.

Excess cortisol also inhibits your body's ability to burn fat for energy. Without an optimal level of fat-burning, sustainable weight loss becomes exceedingly difficult.

 The bottom line is to set aside ME time for deep breathing in order to keep your cortisol levels as low as possible! **Breathe deeply, as if your life depends on it.**

6/

YOU ARE FULLY EQUIPPED

Keep this in mind: you are an unlimited pharmacy of potency. Everything that you need is within you right now. All of the essential mental chemicals and neuro-transmitters that you will ever need are already within your body and brain.

I used to enjoy getting high. You know, finding happiness from external substances. I chased that elusive feeling of ecstasy, and I actually did attain it with Ecstasy. The feeling, however, was short-lived and synthetic; it wasn't pure joy or happiness. It was ephemeral, and it left me feeling empty. On Ecstasy, I enjoyed the ride, but then, soon after, came crashing down, and felt even more depressed, miserable, and worthless.

Drugs did teach me a lot about myself, however. I learned that we all have our limits. And after I ended up in the Emergency Room a few times, I also learned that they are deadly. In addition—and maybe most important—as a result of all of the drugs that I did, experiences that I had, and lows that I felt, I've really come to learn that the natural high of being alive and grateful, living in the moment, and having a clear mind, is the most powerful high of all!

I have found that all of the drugs in the world cannot compare with the human experience. But I learned that lesson the hard way, through 10 years of experimenting with and altering my brain.

All of the drugs that I did were part of my search for happiness. Drugs make you feel temporarily light and carefree; they eliminate your thoughts. But instead of rising above thought, you go beneath it. You use substances to block out your thinking mind in order to feel at one with yourself. When you drink alcohol, you reduce your thoughts and sink below your normal state of consciousness; if you drink enough, you'll even go fully unconscious. That is why alcohol is also called "spirit": when people drink it, they often feel more spiritual, more alive, and more open. But that is an illusion. When you drink, you block yourself out; when you stop, you wake up blurry with a wicked hangover.

Why should we rely on external substances for happiness?

Let's return to my original statement. Everything that YOU need is already within YOU. Once you realize that, you can tap into your own amazing pharmaceutical database. You don't require any illicit toxic substances in your body in order to be happy.

How can you tap into this database and change yourself?

One of the fastest ways to change your beliefs is through your subconscious mind. Your subconscious mind is extremely powerful, and it is, in a sense, like an iceberg. Your conscious mind is the tip of the iceberg, and the subconscious mind is the large, deep, true area where you exist. Your subconscious mind is when you go to sleep and have dreams, and also when you're in a shitty mood and don't know why. Your subconscious mind is constantly talking to you. When you take your ME time, you're just listening to your subconscious mind.

A constant stream of thoughts circulates through your head and feelings. You often don't realize that they're there, however, unless you listen to them or bring them out on paper.

One of the first ways to positively affect your subconscious mind is to listen to it. Here's how:

1. **Simply observe your mind.** This is best done in a closed room where you can just sit and listen. Listen to the chatter; listen to the thoughts. The more that you listen throughout the day, the more you will realize what

tapes are playing, all by themselves, in the background of your thoughts.

2. **Write them out.** Whatever thoughts you have, write them down on paper. If you notice a belief that you feel is irrational, write that down, too. Only when you write it down will you see it for what it truly is.

3. **Talk to people.** Tell others around you what is on your mind: share, vent, and express yourself. When you tell someone else your thoughts, that person can let you know if they're real, or just a figment of your imagination. While you express and open up to the depths of your subconscious mind, you will also realize which of your beliefs and thoughts are helpful or hurtful to you.

The one way that I changed my beliefs was through the use of **affirmations**. I know that it sounds hokey and too good to be true but, actually, affirmations do affect your subconscious.

Through my research, I've come to find that there is a lapse between your conscious conversations and your subconscious mind. It's not that you just say to yourself, "I am happy, I am happy, I am happy," and, instantly, you become happy. Rather, it's a delayed response.

If you say "I am happy, I am happy, I am happy," eventually the message will seep into your subconscious mind and affect your beliefs. However, like I said, it doesn't happen instantly. So, imagine if you're at the top of the iceberg, yelling. It takes some time before the sound travels deep down inside the core of the iceberg, and penetrates into your conscious mind. Think of it as putting in a request, and then having it fulfilled after a certain amount of time.

Also, notice how I said "I am happy" in the present tense.

I said, ***"I am happy."***

Stating any affirmation in the present tense is always more powerful than saying, for example, "*I want to be happy*," or "*I don't want to be upset*." By contrast, when you say "**I am happy**," you believe it to be your current mood.

If you say, "I want to be happy," you kind of don't feel like you *are* happy; that gets communicated to the subconscious mind. So, instead, if you want to drive it deeper, declare your desired outcome in the present moment. Say, "I am Happy **Now!**"

When you make a conscious statement like that, it's almost as though you don't believe it at first. ***That*** is very powerful. That's where your subconscious resides: it is your deep-down core belief that what you currently *have* is working for you.

Another powerful type of affirmation involves asking yourself a question using the outcome *in the present tense.* For example, say I'm feeling down. I could pose this question:

"Why am I so happy right now?"

This then forces my mind to create evidence for why I should be happy. I will think of the many positive aspects of my life, for example, including things for which I'm grateful and the people whom I love. In turn, my mind becomes flooded with reasons for **why I <u>should</u> be happy.** As those reasons seep into my subconscious, I will shift into a chipper mood soon thereafter.

In addition to the positive effects of affirmations, I also discovered that writing down my goals and reading them out loud first thing each morning was very powerful. Your subconscious is at its most receptive when you first wake up, and right before you go to sleep at night. Those two times of day are very important for "putting in the order" to your conscious mind.

So, first thing in the morning and just before sleep are powerful, receptive times to influence your subconscious. I keep a journal by my bedside, and write in it every day. I write about my activities, and all of the good things that happened throughout my day. I write about the various things that I'm grateful for, plus the lessons that I learned, and the things I have done badly. Then, I ask myself, what can I do better?

I also read my goals out loud in the present tense, and focus on my affirmations. I think about how grateful I am, and this gratitude allows me to realize that I am exactly where I should be. I don't need or lack for anything. I have all that I need within me right now. This gives me peace of mind to know that I am fully equipped for whatever life presents me.

As an exercise, spend one day writing out your conscious thoughts. Carry around a small note pad, and observe your inner dialogue. Write down every thought that comes up. Bring it to the foreground. This will be a huge eye-opener. You'll become so much more aware of your daily mental chatter. Your thoughts will seem to increase in volume, and make themselves more apparent.

What I have discovered is that the conversations we have with ourselves are mostly negative and false. Most are not true in the slightest bit, so they undermine us, which creates more stress in our lives. A wise man once said, "All Progress starts with the Truth." I must admit, I felt a little down, once I realized how badly I talk to myself. But the more that I watched my thoughts, the more I was able to look at my inner critic, and re-frame it with the truth.

I urge you try this for just one day. Maintain a discipline of simply writing down all of your self-limiting beliefs. Really see and record your inner dialogue. Once these thoughts come to the surface, you too will realize how much you're stressing yourself out and spiking your cortisol levels.

Once, I watched a video about how raw diamonds are mined. It was fascinating to see how the many layers were stripped away in order to find a diamond's core and maximum brilliance. This reminded me of the layers that we, too, must strip away in order to become better.

Remember how I discussed all of the times that we **add** things into our lives in our quest to become happier? And how strongly I believe that, instead, we need to **subtract** those things that hold us back?

We need to simplify in order to multiply.

The biggest things that hold you back are your limiting beliefs. They come from your inner critic, who tells you constantly that "you're not good enough." Your critic compares what you're doing, currently, with unrealistic or unachievable expectations. Your inner voice can constantly bring you down.

So, do you know what you have to do?

Tell that voice to Shut the F* Up, because it Ain't Helping You!

All that voice does is slow you down.

What I am asking of you here is that you make an effort to become more aware. Simply listen to your inner dialogue. Once you do, you'll be shocked at how much you and your thoughts make you suffer.

I ask that you become aware of it, but remember: don't judge it. Rather, observe it as if it's an annoying little voice that's there to make you realize what's important in your life. The reality is that, if anything upsets you, it means that you value it. It's a sign that you should take it more seriously.

You'll soon realize that you're telling yourself stories that simply aren't true. When you focus on **facts** rather than **fantasy**, you will begin to peel away those limiting beliefs.

Then, an entirely new world will open up, and your heart will fill with gratitude. It is only when you feel grateful that you realize that the stories you tell yourself are nonsense. Once you become aware of them, you'll be able to decrease your stress, cortisol, and cravings, plus you'll be able to lose weight at a much faster pace.

7/

OBSERVE YOUR CHATTERING MIND

"Protect yourself from your own Thoughts."
—Rumi

You are your own worst enemy. The sooner that you realize this, the sooner you will achieve success. Every single day, you have thousands of thoughts which create a mental dialogue that either helps or hurts you.

When things occur in your life, you create stories to make sense of every experience. Whether they are good stories or bad is not important because, in reality, there is no good or bad. **Thinking** makes itself the judge of things. All events are neutral; however, we don't like neutral.

We are, in essence, problem-solving machines, always looking for problems to solve. This, in fact, helped our ancestors, because we used to live in places with vast danger and many threats. Our advanced, problem-solving mind allowed our ancestors to survive in those turbulent times, and to pass on to us genes that became a strong, successful next generation.

Although our civilization and environment has greatly improved, we still have a tendency to look for problems to solve, and for dangers to overcome. That is why our thinking mind runs constantly. It generates an incessant stream of chatter that runs 24/7. Even when you're sleeping, it still does not shut off.

If you listen to it, you'll realize that, most of the time, it's not talking to you in a positive way. So you must observe your thoughts as much as possible.

Soon after you begin this careful and consistent observation, you will understand that being more optimistic will have a dramatic effect on helping you to obtain your fitness goals.

That's why I love to maintain an optimistic outlook in my life. I focus on taking in only positive types of media. I read lots of books that elevate my mind, giving my subconscious plenty of raw materials that help me to see the world in a positive way. I refuse to watch the news, and don't participate in gossip or negative conversations.

Think of it like the computer term "GIGO." **Garbage in, Garbage out**. If you allow negativity into your life, your outlook will become pessimistic, and is certain to affect your mind/body in a detrimental way.

Once, when I was at the park near my house, I noticed a bunch of people walking backwards towards me. A petite, mean-looking woman with a white lab coat was with them walking normally, and guiding them with her hands behind her back.

As they got closer, they seemed to be from a mental institution, and the woman was most likely their aide. I wasn't sure if she was doing an exercise with them, or was just bored, and made them walk backwards to keep herself entertained.

As they passed by me they were all smiling, excited as hell, with their arms flailing about. Their eyes were soft and exuded an inner glow. They all looked to be having the time of their lives, squealing with joy!

They were having so much fun that I even thought about getting up and moon walking. I can't remember the last time I did that!

I decided not to, because the people in the park would probably have thought that I had strayed from the pack of handicapped people. Somebody probably would of grabbed my hand and walked me back to the aide. I didn't feel like explaining myself.

They had great difficulty backwards walking, too. It's challenging enough to walk normally on grass when you're mentally impaired, especially with all the sticks and dog crap. So this was quite a unique task for them.

I was impressed by their determination.

As they continued on, I thought about life, and how we look backwards and compare our future to every past experience. When we start a new venture, we think about a past risk we took. Getting into a relationship, we always think about our ex, and compare him or her to our current companion.

Even starting a diet becomes dreadful when we think about how miserable we felt on the last one. Our past experiences usually dictate our future decisions.

In reality, it's all nonsense, and a severe limitation towards our destined path.

Every single moment is a clean slate with a plethora of possibilities. It's foolish to compare our past, or make a decision in tune with the past.

When we dwell constantly on our prior experiences, we restrict ourselves from the opportunities that lie ahead in our future. Especially with a negative experience, we replay it over and over again, like an annoying rerun.

I mean, how can you move forward when you keep looking back on your past, and labeling it based on prior experiences? When you do that, you turn your back on the Awesomeness that wants to come into your Life.

The past is like the rear-view mirror in your car: it's good to glance back here and there, but stare too long, and you'll miss what's right in front of you.

The bottom line is, nobody gets to live life backwards. You must look ahead with eyes wide open and a heart full of hope.

Every moment is a gift full of infinite possibilities.

Your Life is like book: you'll never enjoy it if you keep re-reading old chapters...

If you're constantly looking back, be prepared to trip on some sticks and land on some dog crap.

8/

TAKE YOUR MIND FOR A WALK

When you read a book, you gain insight. That insight stays in your mind forever. It lies dormant in your memory bank, constantly haunting you if you aren't doing anything with it. However, when you absorb that idea and allow it to take its course in the physical world, all of a sudden you gain power. You gain power of insight and discipline; in addition, you're empowered by the fact that you're acting upon something that you believe in; something that will improve the quality of your life.

One fascinating insight that I gained by watching a very interesting scientific documentary about dementia, cognitive decline, memory loss, and Alzheimer's (which has always been a big fear of mine) was that simply exercising for 20 minutes, three times a week as a minimum, has a tremendous effect on your overall energy, happiness, and state of mind.

Before grasping some of these mindfulness techniques, I was always thinking about my future, or my parents' future, or the futures of my loved ones and friends. Our brains are very powerful and complex; everything exists inside of them. Everything that we've learned can be found in our brains, including our experiences, our wisdom, and, most importantly, our personality. My biggest fear was always that I might lose all of that.

I was really fearful that I could *lose* all of these years of hard work, discipline, studying, learning, and understanding of the world, as well as, all of my memories, connections, and friendships. My biggest fear was that I could possibly lose track of "Who I am."

When I watched that documentary, I thought about my own loved ones going through the same sort of mental breakdown that is brought on by dementia or Alzheimer's. It would be so heartbreaking to speak with your mother and discover that she didn't know who you were. If she were to lose her memory to the point where I was nothing but a stranger to her, all of those years of love, connection, and deep bonding would be taken away from us both.

Memories are very powerful. They are personal stories and connections to our past. So, rather than go off into a deeper tangent about how scary it would be to "lose your mind," I've looked instead at studies that were done on the elderly in order to determine what it is that

helped improve cognitive events. The test subjects were given exercises where they did crossword puzzles, played cards, and even read complicated literature. The study found that, throughout every test, the most powerful tool for preventing cognitive decline was actually **exercise**.

It was interesting to learn that a simple 20 minute walk is more powerful than any mental strategy for improving your cognitive function. Sending oxygen-rich blood into your brain and keeping all of the vessels pumping and running at full capacity will do more to help your memory and brain power than hours and hours of mental strategy. Prior to the prevalent application of antidepressants, doctors used to prescribe a simple walk outside as a popular treatment for depression. Keeping in good physical shape is still a prime component of maintaining a healthy mind, happiness, and a high level of motivation.

I'm not a huge fan of jogging. Instead, throughout the course of my many injuries over the years, I have elected to go for long, brisk walks. I walk at a fast pace, like I'm late for a meeting. This adds a tremendous benefit to my brain, but also gives me peace of mind, and opens me up to taking in many bits of information. It's one thing to sit in a room enclosed by four walls; it's entirely different to walk out in the world, and then take in the sights, sounds, feelings, and smells. When you walk, your senses are inundated with many pieces of stimulating information from the world around you.

When I walk, I fully engage myself with the present moment. I act like I'm an alien from another planet as I listen to music on my iPod or look at trees, cars, and streets. I try to see them as though for the first time, with wonder and awe. I give nothing labels or identities. I just say, "Oh, that's a tree. I see those all the time." I look in awe at its branches, the textures and colors, and wonder at the many long years it took for any given tree to grow into the masterpiece that it is.

Everything around you is beautiful and epic. It's only your own mind that labels something as less, or that gives something an identity that takes away from its greatness. Once you realize this, you can see a simple tree as a masterpiece.

When you *do* look at a simple tree as a masterpiece, you will swiftly realize that *everything in life is a masterpiece,* and everything can have a sense of wonder, awe, and beauty about it. On the other hand, only your mind can reduce things to seeming simple, banal, or redundant.

9/

NEVER A FAILURE, ALWAYS A LESSON

You can either look at the world in awe and beauty, appreciating it as an unfolding masterpiece of amazing moments, or you can look at it as a dreary place with the same old things in it, that occupy space without any meaning.

When you look at the world in awe, you are bound to look at your life in that way, as well.

When you look at the world with a negative mind set, however, and see it as limited and small, dark and dreary, you will habituate your mind to seeing your life as very limited, as well. You will start to think that people are out to get you. You will believe that you're unlucky, and that *everything* bad happens to <u>you</u>. You'll start to take personally the many random daily acts that occur, like parking tickets or bad news, accidents, health conditions, and other incidents that people consider to be negative.

But what if I told you this: **there are no negative situations**. Things are just facts; mere facts. Through our own observation, we make things "heaven" and "hell" by the way in which we label and identify them. *We* make things personal and assume things.

The simple act of getting a parking ticket—walking to your car and seeing a ticket on your windshield—can make you feel like the world is out to get you. Like you are the only unlucky person with that parking ticket, and clearly the universe is conspiring in order to make your life a living hell.

You can feel like you are being punished. "Why me?" you ask, when you look around and see that no other car has a ticket like yours. Suddenly, you think the simple act of going shopping is going to cost you a lot more because of that parking ticket. You begin to develop the "poor me" mindset, full of negative thoughts and stupid labels.

In this syndrome, you look at the world as a dark and dreary place, limited by the fact that money is going out of your pocket. You feel like less of a person … I know that sounds crazy! But these are the normal thoughts that a person has when we look at something and see it as a kind of "hell."

On the other hand, making a situation into "heaven" requires more work. Unfortunately, it's a lot easier to get into a negative mind set, to worry and be anxious when certain things occur, rather than look at it from a "heaven" point of view. But, in truth, it's just a lesson. In fact, there are **no failures, only lessons**.

You can look at that same parking ticket and realize that this is a lesson because you made a mistake. You *could* say, "Thank God I got this ticket. It's money that I'll gladly pay. Plus, the fines go to support the city, and will add quality to someone else's life, as well as, my own. In addition, I'm <u>not</u> the only person that got a ticket. It's *not just about me!*"

Let's look at another example. What if, instead of getting a parking ticket, your car didn't start? Or what if your car got stolen? That would cost a lot more than the measly ticket. What about the idea that, maybe, had you not found that ticket and stopped to read it for a few minutes, you might have driven off and gotten into a bad collision or fatal car accident!

I know it may sound crazy to create those alternative scenarios in your mind. But instead of generating negative stories that make something into a "hell" by taking it personally, why not put "heavenly" stories into your mind, instead? Why not try and make sense out of what happens, rather than see the world as limited? When you do that, you will see the world as abundant. You will see the world as **conspiring to <u>help</u> you.** You will feel a force leading you on the right path, and realize that everything is relative.

I think that relativity is a very important concept, and one which doesn't often receive much focus. Everything is relative, isn't it? A parking ticket that costs $50 may seem like a lot when you compare it to zero. Taking $50 out of your bank account or having to spend money that you don't have, when your debts are accumulating, can seem like a big setback. But $50 compared to finding that your car won't start, so that you have to tow it to a mechanic who may charge you $500, seems much less!

Also, the fact that the $50 upsets you, but could have saved you from driving into a fatal accident, makes the amount seem miniscule. In relativity, there's always something worse that could happen.

That's what helped me. Basically, when bad things happen, I urge you to be thankful because thinking of some worse-case scenarios can bring new perspective to any "minor setback."

There are so many worse-case scenarios to consider. For example, think of bigger financial burdens, sickness or injury, or even traumatic, life-changing events, like the loss of a limb or the death of a loved one. Even consider the worst-case scenario: your own death.

If you're alive and breathing and overcame that set-back, then all of a sudden that little ticket ain't so bad, is it?

Of course, these mental strategies are not easy to implement, and don't happen automatically. Anything worthwhile requires work and effort. The same goes for the physical aspect of being in shape, looking and feeling good. It doesn't happen automatically. When we are overweight, diseased, or tired all the time, we need to try and create good habits. If we didn't brush our teeth every day, our teeth would decay and fall out over time, right? The same thing applies to your mind. It requires daily discipline, good habits, and regular exercise. Physical improvements require work just as much as the mental ones do.

In order to maximize your peak physical state, make sure that you are always aware of your physical being. That means, your posture, the way you walk, and even your facial expressions. Your physical mannerisms are important because they tend to affect your mental state. You need to pay attention to the physical aspects of your everyday movement.

You may say to yourself, "Wow, this is a lot of work. I can't possibly think about so many things. This is ridiculous. I am not a robot!"

Well, remember: your other choice is to think about your past or to have anxiety about your future. Unless you start to notice your repetitive thoughts, like I stated in the beginning, you will always have incessant pointless thinking that causes more harm than good.

Focus your attention on the present moment and on your physical senses. This will bring more clarity to your mind. It will also add more power to the moment, thus give you more energy and a better external representation to the outside world.

Just think about it: when a person walks into a room with their head held high, perfectly erect posture, smiling, confident and happy, don't you respond differently than to someone who arrives looking down, with a slouched posture and slight frown on his or her face? Which one of these people would you be more apt to interact with? Which one looks more attractive to you? Which commands more attention?

There you have it. Your goal is to **be that person who walks around at a peak state** wherever you go. Not just for other people. Do this when you're alone as well, and when you're with your significant other, or even if you're in the middle of nowhere, walking by yourself.

Walk each step with your head held high as if every part of your foot is touching the ground. Feel the sensations of the world moving beneath your feet. You are a special person, and each step that you take is helping the Earth's rotation. As you walk, hold your head up high, ready for the world, with a slight smirk on your face. Feel content and present. I know that this may seem like delusional thinking; however, you are meant to be in this state.

Walking with full confidence and full presence is your **natural essence.** The more that you focus on your surroundings and internal physical feelings, the more energy and alertness you will have. You'll realize that you have more power, and you'll call more attention to yourself from others. You will look like a person who is at one with themselves.

Another fascinating factor; when you are focused on clearing your mind, and when you pay attention to your physical sensations, you think much less, so that incessant stream of useless thoughts isn't circulating. You're at peace. In a sense, you are like a blank slate, receptive to the present moment. And that is powerful.

10/

THE POWER OF YOUR TRUE ESSENCE

When a person makes a comment, your mind operates quickly in order to react with an answer. Also, when you're talking to somebody, you're fully engaged in their conversation, listening wholeheartedly with every word, not judging. You want to give great answers, too, but if you are thinking about something else, you are not being fair to them.

It is selfish to have a person speak to you while only a small percentage of your attention is on their words. In that case, the other parts of your attention are in your own mind, which is pointless thinking. Think about how much funnier you would be if you were in the moment, and somebody made a comment. You could respond with a witty remark.

When people are around you, they will generally enjoy you more when you're calm, present, and caring. So, practice this as much as you can. Like anything else, it's a step-by-step process. Don't expect yourself to be able to do this consistently, 24 hours a day. It takes time and planning.

I focus on a reminder system for myself. Sometimes, I put a simple stamp on my hand to remind me. Others put a rubber band around their wrist, and give it a gentle snap to bring them back into the moment. Whatever your method is of bringing your mind back to the present moment, the more that you practice it, the more it will become habitual. I have now done this practice for so long that, every time I stand upright, I realize I have great physical power whenever I am less focused on my mind and more focused on the present moment and the world around me.

This is true power, and again, it is **your true essence**. The busy brain that you have was useful thousands of years ago. The only danger that you are confronted with nowadays in our safe world, however, is yourself.

11/

CHANGE YOUR THOUGHTS, CHANGE YOUR MOOD

One of the most profound exercises that I've found came from a best-selling book about treating depression and anxiety. It is called "Feeling Good" by David M. Burns, and really changed my whole paradigm on depression and anxiety.

It's based on **cognitive behavioral therapy**, which is a type of psychological therapy that focuses on a person's thoughts and outlook. I find it interesting because cognitive behavioral therapy, or CBT, has been shown to decrease a person's mental illness without any drugs or aggressive methods. What is fascinating is that CBT has a much higher success rate for treating depression and anxiety when compared with more aggressive treatments like medication or other interventions.

Rather than delve into the full science behind CBT and how effective it is, I'm going to give you the Cliff

Notes version of it, and teach you a very powerful exercise. CBT subscribes to the philosophy that your thoughts are the cause of mental illness. So, by changing your thoughts, you improve your mood.

The major cause of all negative emotion is irrational thinking. What I mean by irrational is **thinking about negative things or circumstances that may never happen.** Our thinking, as I stated earlier, is more harmful than beneficial. We tend to dwell on our past or think about our future. When it comes to the past, you relive traumatic experiences that happened to you. Alternately, you are anxious about future events that usually never happen.

When we are thinking irrationally, stuck in past and future moments, we waste precious time. What irrational thinking does is, it creates untrue stories that we tend to believe. Many times, this happens on an unconscious level, where your mind thinks irrational thoughts, erratically. Cognitive behavioral therapy teaches you how to identify your irrational thoughts so that you realize which ones aren't true.

When you realize that most all of them are not true, these thoughts lose their power to affect you or make you upset. Instead, you replace them with the truth. The truth really does set you free, especially when you compare it to your irrational thoughts.

*****

Usually, when we are upset, a call to a loved one makes us feel better.

Let's say that you're having a rough day at work. You call up a friend or loved one, and share how you're in a stressful circumstance. The incident involves how your boss made you upset. Maybe everything that your boss said made you feel depressed and anxious about the future, or suggested to you that you're not good enough or even a full-on failure. The day may have been so bad that you are afraid that you may lose your job, which would inevitably result (*in your **mind***) to becoming broke and homeless. It's just a few short steps until you're starving on the cold streets, begging for change!

Usually, if your friend cares about you, he or she will set you straight. They'll remind you that whatever happened was merely your boss' opinion. In addition, maybe your boss was just having a bad day and took it out on you: whatever they said doesn't mean that <u>you</u> are a failure. It certainly does not mean that you are any less capable or competent a person, so this incident <u>should not be taken personally</u>.

It is not a "fact"—and very unlikely—that you will be homeless, destitute, and starving on the streets. Hopefully your friend will then remind you of positive things, in order to cheer you up and make you feel better. In fact, the interaction between you two could be very helpful and beneficial. It is a positive practice for you to share deep thoughts about yourself and specific, irrational fears that are not true in the least.

When you express the details of your stressful fantasy to your friend, you will come to realize that everything that you have described is completely irrational. You can even see that the "fact" that you are worrying about or the fear that you have generated is causing more harm to you than the actual experience itself.

This conversation will also cause you to be very honest and truthful with your friend, to share your deepest and darkest thoughts. Many times, it's somewhat difficult to share things that you're really feeling, and to be completely honest. If you're good at it, that's great; I commend you. In general, however, it's tough for us to be completely honest with people. But the more that you do it; the better able they'll be to show that they are good-hearted and caring.

If you don't have a close friend, or if you don't feel like sharing a specific thought, you can actually use this powerful CBT technique by yourself.

The technique is called the **double column exercise**.

Even though we are intelligent, we still believe in our irrational thoughts. They circulate in our minds and repeat themselves over and over. It is easy to believe our unquestioned thoughts.

But when we do, we allow these harmful thoughts to affect our moods. We severely limit ourselves when we believe them. This causes unnecessary pain and suffering. So, instead of going to a therapist and getting CBT therapy by a professional, you can also do this method on your own.

That is not to say that I want you to avoid going to a therapist! There are certain cases where the severity of a person's mental illness requires a psychologist. However, you should try this exercise on your own the next time that you're feeling down, or if you're anxious about a specific event.

The **double column exercise** is very simply the act of expressing your irrational thoughts. This can be done in two ways. In the first, you call up a friend and vent all of the thoughts that you are thinking; many times, your friend will reassure you of the truth, and once you realize that your irrational thoughts are not true and have no power, their negative effects on you will be reduced.

The other option is to do the double column exercise. It, too, shows you how irrational your thoughts can be. Your thoughts are like your computer's operating system. They dictate constantly what is true and what is not. But when you take those thoughts out of your mind and put them down on paper, you expose them to the truth. It is then possible for you to realize that they are false, that they are making you upset, and that they are putting you in a negative state of mind.

This exercise is simple. Take a blank sheet of paper and draw a line down the middle, from top to bottom. Title the left column "IRRATIONAL THOUGHTS," and the right column, "FACTS."

First, on the left side, write down each one of your irrational thoughts, no matter how crazy they sound. Then, on the right, write the specific facts that prove that your irrational thoughts *aren't* true.

Personally, I use the double column exercise any time that I feel down and out, or when I'm anxious about a specific event. It is not always easy to sit down and do this exercise, expressing yourself this way. However, it's worth making the effort because it is extremely powerful. It shines the light of truth on your erratic thinking. Once I complete the exercise, I always feel like my mind is made clear, and I'm able to realize what the truth really is.

The bottom line is this: most of the time, you are thinking about things that never happen or won't occur in the way that you think about them. The worst things happen *in your mind,* rather than in real life! By becoming aware of your irrational thoughts and how they affect your moods, you will develop a much better understanding of yourself. This will put you on the right path to thinking about the truth.

12/

PRACTICAL TIPS

Tense Up

The next time that you think about straying from your diet, **clench your fists**! Researchers have discovered that people who tense their muscles when tempted by fattening foods have more self-control than those who don't.

So, try to squeeze the handles of your shopping cart as you walk down the supermarket aisles whenever you see your favorite snack. Or flex your feet when you're holding the dessert menu in a restaurant.

Remember, this only works at the moment of decision! But after you do it a few times, you'll notice that, every time you "Clench your Fists," an anchor is created that reminds you to have self-control.

<u>More practical eating tips</u>:

1. Eat when you are hungry.

2. Eat sitting down in a calm environment.

3. Eat without distractions. Distractions include radio, television, newspapers, books, or intense conversation.

4. Eat very slowly with enjoyment and pleasure.

Whether you weigh 350 pounds or 150 pounds, when you are not hungry, you are using food as a drug, grappling with boredom. Food can become a middleman that you cling to. It acts as the means to your end of altering your emotions, of making yourself numb, of creating a secondary problem, while the original problem becomes too uncomfortable.

Comfort Foods

Why is macaroni and cheese a comfort food for some people, while meatloaf is comfort food for others? Most people can't tell you.

Comfort food connections are almost always formed subconsciously. Past associations are the most common reasons for a food becoming a comfort food. Some of these associations can be linked to specific individuals or events. They're also connected with feelings that you like to recall or want to recapture.

In some cases, these are vivid experiences that you flash on when thinking, tasting or smelling certain foods. These memories evoke feelings of safety, love, appreciation, control, and empowerment.

The psychological need for the feeling pulls you towards those foods. While some people are drawn to comfort food because of their past associations, others may be drawn towards the same food because they identify with it personally.

Make comfort foods more comforting. Never say to yourself, "I will never eat pizza or cookies again in my life."

If you say that, you will be destined for failure. Comfort foods help make life enjoyable. The key is to learn how to have your cake and eat it too. Don't deprive yourself. Keep your comfort foods, but eat them in smaller amounts when you have "cheat meals."

To find out why you crave comfort foods, ask yourself these questions.

1. Why do you like it so much?

2. When do you usually crave it, and why is it comforting?

For example, my comfort food is Chunky Peanut Butter.

1. **Why do you like it so much?** The contrasting sweet and salty elements taste good, and the thick and creamy texture is very filling. I love being FULL!

2. **When do you usually crave it, and why is it comforting?** I usually crave chunky peanut butter at night after dinner. It always fills me up, and I feel happy and relaxed afterwards. Eating it brings back memories of being a kid, and makes me feel cozy and safe.

The problem is that I usually have 4 tablespoons at a time, and that's 400 calories—YIKES! Sadly, I'm addicted to chunky peanut butter, and actually banned it from my house. Whenever I get into an emotional eating pattern, I start to stick my spoon in the jar until my belly gets nice and full.

I can't control myself to only have 1 spoonful. Since then, I've replaced my chunky peanut butter with a lower-calorie version that has the same creamy texture. It still makes me feel warm and fuzzy.

Craving VS Hunger Cheat Sheet

What are you hungry for? Do you want a Snicker's bar, or do you really want a hug?

I read a book called "Think Thin Be Thin," and it offered the following Cheat Sheet to let you know if you're responding to physical hunger, or feeding a deeper craving need.

Physical hunger builds gradually. A Craving develops suddenly.

Physical hunger strikes below the neck, e.g. a growling stomach. A Craving: above the neck, e.g. a taste for ice cream.

Physical hunger occurs several hours after a meal. A Craving is unrelated to time.

Physical hunger goes away when full. A Craving persists despite fullness.

Physical hunger eating leads to a feeling of satisfaction. Craving eating leads to guilt and shame.

Physical Hunger Signals

Being aware of your body's physical hunger signals can help give you the confidence you need to satisfy your food cravings. Hunger signals can come from your stomach, informing you that it is empty, or from your brain, letting you know that it is lacking in an energy supply.

Signals from your stomach may include growls, pangs, or hollow feelings. Signals from your brain may include fogginess, lack of concentration, headache, or fatigue.

If you still are not sure whether you are truly hungry, try using the following **Hunger/Fullness Rating Scale.**

- 10 - Absolutely, positively stuffed
- 9 - So full that it hurts
- 8 - Very full and bloated
- 7 - Starting to feel uncomfortable
- 6 - Slightly overeaten
- 5 - Perfectly comfortable
- 4 - First signals that your body needs food
- 3 - Strong signals to eat
- 2 - Very hungry, irritable
- 1 - Extreme hunger, dizziness

Eating Triggers

Many things can trigger our desire to eat: the aroma of food, the sight of a favorite food, a commercial on television, or just knowing that there are sweets in the house.

I'm an emotional eater, and my cravings are always triggered when I'm in a bad mood.

The habit of eating while watching television can make television an eating trigger.

That is why **Awareness is key**. Recognizing what triggers your cravings is the first step in learning to control them.

Portion Control

In the past, one of my biggest issues was eating too quickly. I devoured my food like a ravenous dog. I would literally eat as if I was in a race to stuff my face. I'd clear my plate faster than a normal person swallowed their first bite. I'm convinced that this caused my chipmunk cheeks throughout those years when I was overweight.

I also had a bad habit of making sure that there wasn't a single morsel of food left on my plate. At times, I would even go so far as to lick the plate ... (Yes, I was that bad!) I was conditioned by my parents to have respect for the have-nots in this world, and not waste any food. I would routinely clear my plate so that I didn't have to throw food away.

Over the years, I made a change. I slowed down my eating, and stopped stuffing my face like a Hungry Hippo. I started to eat intuitively; I ate more slowly and paid more attention to my internal hunger cues.

When you eat more slowly, there is actually a better chance that your food will be used as energy, rather than stored as FAT.

Research has shown that if you eat a meal in 10 minutes, you will eat on average 100 calories more than if you ate the same meal over a 30-minute time span.

It's much better to savor each bite and slowly focus on chewing. Allow your taste buds to experience every intricate sensation in the process of eating.

I noticed that, when I did this, I ate far less, and walked away from my meals feeling satisfied, rather than feeling sluggish and swollen.

As I mentioned, it takes approximately 20 minutes for your stomach to sense that it is full, so eating your meal over a 30-minute time period allows you to stop when the body senses its level of fullness.

Essentially, people who eat very quickly do not take advantage of the body's natural satiety indicator.

Also: see how much less you eat by **using chop sticks** instead of a fork or spoon! Not only will this take you longer to eat, you will also become a chop stick pro!

Remember, the longer you take to eat, the faster you will feel full, and the fewer calories you will consume overall.

Here are some more tips:

When you plate your food, always **use the small-size dinnerware**. For example, try using dessert plates instead of big massive food plates.

We always try to fill our plates, but if you use the smaller ones, they become filled faster with food.

Imagine your normal meal on a huge plate. Your eyes will deceive you into thinking that your portion is too small.

When you drink your beverages, try to **use smaller, more slender glasses.**

By using smaller slender glasses, you can fake out your mind that you already had an entire glass of soda or juice, when in reality you only had a half of a glass.

13/

THE SUMMER I FOUND MY SIX PACK

One weekend, I was cleaning out my attic. As I sorted through old clothes and boxes, reminiscing, I came across a small tattered album of photos. It brought back many memories of my youth. One picture in particular reminded me of a life-changing experience that I want to share with you.

It was from the summer that I found my six-pack!

As I've shared, I was overweight for most of my life. This was really tough on me, both physically and mentally.

Back then, never in my wildest dreams did I think that I would ever have a 6-pack.

For as long as I could remember, in fact, having ripped abs seemed like an impossible goal. I've since come to realize that we don't make major changes in our life until we hit rock bottom. And I did hit rock bottom.

That one summer, I really hit a rough spot. There I was: fat, unhappy, and insecure as I drove to the beach with my girlfriend at the time.

I firmly believe that there's a correlation between the number of years in a relationship and the inches around your waist ... LOL! Being comfortable in that relationship, I had let myself go. I was in **no** shape to go to the beach and strip down to a bathing suit.

I remember having anxiety just driving there. My nerves began to take over as I got in my car. I sat in the driver's seat and could feel my gut flowing over the top of my seat belt buckle. It made me nauseous.

I had a nice set of B-cup man boobs, too, that would have made a teenage girl jealous. No matter what kind of shirt I wore, those things would stick out and command attention. I *hated* my man boobs. They were the obvious sign of being obese. I first grew them as a teen, when my hormones were running wild. During those formative years, when your body fat stays high for a long period of time, it causes your body to pump out more estrogen. Hence, it was slowly turning me into a Dolly Parton.

The worst part of being overweight, for me, was having a permanently bloated face. My cheeks have been chubby since the day I was born, and my aunts loved to squeeze them! You know how embarrassing that is, at least for a boy. No matter what I did, those cheeks always stared back at me in the mirror. Even worse, when I looked in pictures, I saw this strange moon-faced dude staring back at me.

I didn't feel like my true self. I felt like the Goodyear blimp, driving to the beach.

There I was, sitting in the driver's seat while my girlfriend sat next to me, wearing a tight basketball jersey that felt like Saran Wrap over my jiggly rolls. I felt so insecure with myself that it radiated out of every pore. My low self-esteem had a huge effect on my relationship at the time.

When we got to the beach, I decided to keep my tank top on. I made an excuse about feeling cold, when in reality I felt embarrassed about how I looked. Even worse, on that particular day I was the only guy at the beach fully clothed. Everybody else frolicked around half-naked like it was nothing.

I felt ashamed whenever a lean guy walked past me with a flat stomach. I kept thinking, "He is *so lucky* to look like that."

I even followed my girlfriend's eyes and felt jealous that she must be staring at every ripped guy around me. I felt inferior the entire time we were there. If I could have, I would have buried my head in the sand!

You know what? It feels good telling you this story because I now realize how much confidence I lacked back then. That day at the beach was extremely painful, and it really made me depressed and upset.

Shortly afterwards, the combination of my insecurity and low self-worth took its toll on our relationship, and it came to an abrupt end. There were other issues in our relationship, but having low self-confidence was the ultimate catalyst.

So there I was, lonely, heartbroken and heavy during the first week of June. I knew that this wasn't the life for me. **Something had to change** because I sure as hell wasn't going to spend my summer ashamed, miserable, and alone in that fat suit I called my body.

No way, José!

I have an extreme mentality, which means that I tend to go all out, if I put my mind to something.

Being obese was one extreme. It represented the sum total of hardly going to the gym, of overeating, and of generally being lazy.

It was time to go for the opposite extreme.

I had worked out and dieted in the past, but never gotten the results that I wanted.

So I said to myself:

"This summer I am going to get myself into the best shape EVER!!"

I was determined to get a six pack. After that miserable day at the beach, trapped in my overweight physique, I set a goal to achieve the opposite extreme.

My *goal was to have a 6-pack on my birthday, Aug 22!* I only had 2 months, but I was on a mission! I was hyped up and motivated, something that I hadn't felt in a very long time.

I got my hands on everything possible in order to learn how to add muscle, burn fat, and shape up my body. I was already a member at a gym, but I wasn't consistent. I decided to go every day, and at least do something while I was there.

I remember feeling this crazy energy at the time, as if I were possessed to make major progress. I knew that, if I wanted a 6-pack in two months, there was no room for error. I had to hire experts who could get me there faster and safer than I could, doing it all by myself. My tunnel vision was on full force, and I was **On A Mission**!

I went and hired the busiest personal trainer at my gym to guide me. Unfortunately, he wasn't certified to give me nutritional advice, so I also hired the best online nutritional guru at the time named Chris. Chris actually taught me a lot about nutrition, and explained much of what I teach today, myself. (Sadly, Chris died a violent death shortly after he coached me. More on this tragedy another time...)

I discovered a great deal about myself that summer, as I spent hours in the gym and made my fitness a priority. I really got to know who I was, where I wanted to go, and all about the body-transformation process. A lot of what I learned then, I still share today with my clients. It has helped me tremendously in my understanding of how the body adds muscle and takes off fat.

I also noticed, as I lost weight each week, my confidence grew. I was beginning to get ALOT more attention from the opposite sex. My man boobs shrank, and my stomach became flatter and tighter. Best of all, my face became more chiseled as my chubby cheeks slowly dissolved!

I was on FIRE!!! No one was stopping me now!

I think that is how I chose the word "*Unstoppable*" to keep me focused and to persevere.

As I got slimmer and saw more progress, I worked even harder, which further accelerated my results! I stayed focused on the nutrition plan that had been prepared for me by my coach, and all I could think about was reaching my goal on my birthday!

As the time drew closer to the big day, I began to feel anxious. I woke up one morning, still groggy, and looked down to see this outline of my abs popping through my belly fat! They were like alien bumps on my stomach.

I was so excited, it almost made me cry!!

I still feel that overwhelming joy today.

There is something truly special about looking down and seeing a flat stomach.

Man, it was a tough two months!

Finally, the Day of Judgment had arrived…

I could feel the empty spaces where mounds of fat used to be. No more hanging belly! No more soft squishy man boobs! And best of all, my face opened up and my eyes seemed brighter. My chipmunk cheeks were gone, and my eyes shone bright where they used to look squinted like a blow fish.

I found me!

Losing all of that weight made me look younger, and gave me an unstoppable feeling like I was on Top of the World!

I REALLY DID IT!!!!

I had the feeling that nothing could ever stop me now!

AUG 22 CAME, AND I HAD A VISIBLE 6-PACK ON MY BIRTHDAY.

Best of all, I had learned so much about myself, in the process of finding my 6 pack. I also learned some great ways to help others do the same.

It's amazing how looking at an old photo can flood your mind with memories of how much your life has changed. That summer will forever remain a milestone in my life.

It's moments like this that have changed my destiny. I am so blessed to have had those tough times turn into blessings.

That summer also made me discover my passion for helping others. It led me to my majoring in exercise, science and nutrition at college, and then to getting my Master's in psychology.

I needed to understand all of the available tools in order to help others reach the same goals that I reached … the Mind Body Solution!

I will never forget how the experiences of losing weight and being at my best made me feel. That specific moment improved my life more than anything that I've gone through. It led me to my purpose.

My purpose is still to help you be at your best! I will do everything in my power to assist you with your fitness goals...

Thanks so much for reading my story, and for allowing me to share this personal part of my life journey with you.

14/

CONCLUSION: THE ABUNDANCE MINDSET

Sometimes I get down on myself because certain things don't live up to my expectations. When I feel down, however, I GIVE to others what I feel is lacking in my life. I know that this sounds crazy, but hear me out...

One of the secrets of getting everything that you want out of life is the simple act of **giving to somebody else**. Now, this may seem like a weird concept, but whatever you feel like you are lacking, try to give it to another person.

If you're in need of money, for example, rather than kill yourself trying to make more, help somebody else make money. Give them an idea, give them a referral, or simply give some money to charity. By no means am I saying that you should give with the idea of wanting something, in return. On the other hand, for those who say that you should ONLY devote your life to helping and giving, well, thumbs up to you. But very few of us are a Mother Theresa.

Basically, you want to add value to the world constantly by giving things that you are passionate about. This constant giving creates a void, which in turn makes people feel indebted to you. They will eventually want to return the favor by helping you or by referring business to you, or maybe even paying you in some way.

You have to focus on **adding as much value** as possible. We are all passionate about certain things, and we've all been gifted with certain qualities, skills, and talents that only we have. Giving and sharing your passions with others will give *you* a powerful sense of purpose. Where can you give certain parts of yourself that will help somebody else?

Let's take a moment here. Let's say that you are passionate, but you _don't_ feel comfortable giving to others. Or maybe you don't have the confidence to give somebody advice or teach somebody something. Well, you can still start with the small act of sharing a powerful, heartfelt, honest compliment with someone.

Personally, I have the simple goal of **giving one compliment a day**. A few simple, loving words expressed at the right time can change the course and meaning of one's entire life...

In fact, I'm here today because certain people believed in me. They lifted me higher than what I thought was possible. Whether they were family, teachers or friends, they created a gap for me to fill. They highlighted the attributes that I had overlooked, and pushed me to be a greater version of myself. I am forever indebted to them, and deeply grateful for their faith in me.

Understanding this, I realized the power of a compliment. It's truly amazing how your words can shape and influence a person's life. A small effort of praise can significantly alter another person's destiny.

Use this same principle towards **love**. If you're feeling lonely, and you feel that nobody is showing you love, hook up one of your friends on a date, or give somebody a loving compliment. Simply help someone else attain what you feel is missing in your life.

By constantly GIVING, you will change your mindset to that of ABUNDANCE.

When you have an abundant belief system, a well of possibilities will flow forever and never end. You have the ability to GIVE to others, and HELP them accomplish their goals. You operate with a sense of gratitude, and you know, deep down inside, that there's more than enough for EVERYONE.

In reality, that familiar needy feeling is nothing more than *scarcity*. Scarcity causes you to see the world as limited, and contributes to your feeling like there's never enough.

I'm not even going to get into the spiritual side of this. Rather, I encourage you to think about how beneficial this is, logically.

To sum it up: If you feel that something is missing in your life, help someone else to achieve it. Give it a try. Even for a day. Try to **GIVE what you Lack** to every single person that you come in contact with, whether it's a compliment, an introduction to someone of value, or simply some help with their struggles.

Focus on giving. That pretty much sums up this entire book! I felt a deep need to share my experiences and my knowledge with others, along with my thoughts.

I have learned how incredibly much these thoughts have helped me. For me *not* to share them would do the world an injustice. That is how this book came to be. I felt this inner urge to share my philosophy with all of you, an urge so great that it compelled me to write a book and share this side of myself.

I want to finish by saying this: **YOU have something within you that wants to be let out,** something that wants and needs to be shared. I am sure that you didn't reach the end of this book without thinking about what you are passionate about, and what you want to give to the world. I'm not just asking you to help me out! Please help society as a whole, by helping someone to become better.

15/

MY GIFT TO YOU!

I want to give you a Gift!

I am offering you a *free weight-loss program* to thank you for reading this book. It will show you how to put into action some of the strategies that have worked for me.

All you need to do is to email me here:

AJMihrzadCoach@gmail.com

I'll respond by emailing you back the program. Please download and try out. Then let me know what you think about it!

I *know* that it will inspire you to adopt the **Mind-Body Solution** with your own skills and abilities, and then to attain your goals.

ALSO, please visit my website: **LifeFuelFit.com**.

There, you can sign up for my eNewsletter where I offer you regular, ongoing health, nutrition, and workout tips, plus encouragement, wisdom, and community. When you subscribe to my content, the energy and benefits of this book continue to ripple out to you and your endeavors. Check it out now!

Also, please join my Facebook Page and share your experiences, putting into practice some of the strategies in this book. I'd love you to make posts anytime on my wall: https://www.facebook.com/LifeFuelFit

And guess what? You can HIRE ME!

I have clients from all over the world. Send me an email for some special information on my services, and let me help you even more, as you attain your mind-body fitness best:

AJMihrzadCoach@gmail.com)

THANK YOU SO MUCH!

-AJ Mihrzad

ABOUT THE AUTHOR

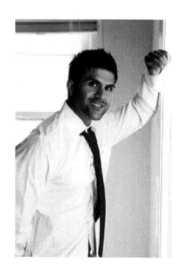

AJ Mihrzad is the owner of Life Fuel Fitness based in Great Neck, New York. LifeFuel Fitness has been Voted the #1 Fitness/Weight-Loss Program in Long Island by the Best of Great Neck Award Program. AJ is also the founder of LifeFuel Supplements, along with fitness software called LeanBuddy. AJ has been featured in Men's Fitness and on Bodybuilding.com.

AJ has a Bachelor of Science degree in exercise science and nutrition as well as a Masters in psychology.

Connect with him on Facebook here:

https://www.facebook.com/LifeFuelFit

Made in the USA
San Bernardino, CA
11 October 2014